Constipation Remedies

Vivek Kamath

ISBN-13 978-1523468546

ACKNOWLEDGEMENT

I am grateful to my mother Late Mrs. Vimala Kamath for giving me the birth because of which I am able to attain this great moment of writing a book on "Constipation Remedies ". My Mother died of Diabetes and Cardiac Aliment way back in November 2006. Today I am able to cure Diabetes, Heart Aliment thru Reiki healing method and many other diseases without Medicines. It was unfortunate that I do not have my mother with me. I am sure her departed soul will now be able to rest in peace today by seeing the achievement of her beloved son. My mother's love and affection was a key for me to attain this position today and instrumental in shaping up my life and destiny. I am very thankful to my mother for giving me this great opportunity to serve the world.

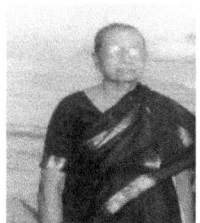

I would like to express my gratitude and heart-full of love to great Reiki Guru and Founder Dr Mikao Usui of Japan.

I would like to thank myself because of my inner strength with which I could able to convert the difficult situations or challenges faced in my life as a great opportunity for learning and always believed that life is a continuous education process. Furthermore, I strongly believed in my life that whatever happens in life it will happen for a good cause and these are based on our good and bad karma/action of past and current life.

CONTENTS

1 Introduction

Background about the Author

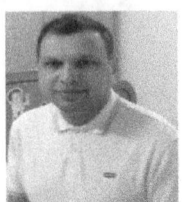

Author Vivek Kamath is an Indian Software Engineer by profession. Author has worked with the world's top International Banks across the globe for nearly 20 years to manage large scale Information Technology (IT) projects. Author is also a Reiki Healing Master Cum Practitioner and Practicing Reiki Healing, Mexican Healing, Crystal Healing, Melchizedek Method of healing from the last 5 years. Author has healed many diabetic patients, blood pressure patients (both high and low blood pressure), Heart Patients (removed the heart blocks), removed kidney stones , cured sinusitis, severe joint pains, constipation, migraines, headaches, insomnia, stomach related problems, diabetic gum problems, skin problems (dry skin, eczema) and chronic nasal allergies, nasal blockages without any medicines. Some of the above treatments have been completed within a week to maximum 1 month duration. Author has intention to help as much as diabetic patients to come out of the disease without any medicines. Author has an intention to build a healing center for diabetic patients across the globe.

For whom was this book prepared?

This book intended for people who are suffering from constipation and piles problem. If in case patients are not able to heal constipation and piles problems with herbal remedies, author has suggested constipation patients to go for an option 2 Healing Cure. There are various Healing methods to heal constipation. Author has mentioned about Reiki Healing in this book.

Author has healed several of his patients who were having chronic constipation and irregular bowel movements. Some of the patients have been completely cured from constipation without any medicines. Author has used distant healing method (Patients can reside far away from the healer) of Reiki to heal some of the patients. Distant healing has been found to be very effective.

2 What is Constipation?

The word **constipation** comes from the Latin *constipare* meaning "to press, crowd together", and from 1400 A.D. Latin *Constipationem*. According to Medilexicon's medical dictionary, constipation is *"A condition in which bowel movements are infrequent or incomplete"*.

Constipation is an irregular bowel syndrome it can mean that you're not passing stool regularly or unable to completely empty your bowel. Constipation occurs when bowel movement become less frequent and difficult. It can affect people at all ages. It can cause your stools to be hard and lumpy, as well as unusually large or small. If it is not treated on time, it could lead to some severe complication such as hemorrhoids(piles) , anal fissures, or fecal impaction.

Digestive System Process

In your digestion process, after eating, food moves through our digestive tract. The body produces digestive enzymes that start to break down food in the mouth. As it moves through your esophagus and stomach, the food becomes liquefied which makes it possible for body to absorb nutrients in it.

Role of Small Intestine

The small intestine, actually absorbs all of the good things from food including protein, carbohydrates, and fats. It also absorbs vitamins and minerals through the walls of the small intestine. And once all the nutrients that can be absorbed have been removed, final part of the metabolism process is left with water and waste.

Role of Large Intestine (Colon)

In the large intestine the water is removed from the waste of food and begins to solidify into what we call feces. As food passes through the large intestine more and more water is removed until you have a bowel movement to release it from the body.

The slower the food moves through your digestive tract, the more water the colon will absorb from food.

Consequently, the feces become dry and hard.
Defecation (emptying the bowels) can become very painful, and in some serious cases there may be symptoms of bowel obstruction. When the constipation is very severe; when the constipation prevents the passage of feces and gas, it is called obstipation. Please see the below diagram on constipation process.

3 Symptoms of Constipation

Below are some of the symptoms of the constipation.

1. Difficulty in Passing stool

2. Opening bowels less than 2 or 3 times a week

3. Hard Dry, Abnormally small or large stool

4. Staining to pass stool

5. Severe Bloating and Abdominal Pain

6. Headache, Bad Taste in Mouth, Nausea and Feeling of Sluggishness

7. Loss of Appetite in some cases

8. Stomach Ache and Cramps

9. Foul-smelling wind and stools

4. Causes of Constipation

1. Dietary Conditions (not having enough fiber, fruits, vegetables and lack of daily consumption of water/fluid in your daily diet)
2. Antacid medicines containing calcium or aluminum
3. Eating a lot of dairy products.
4. Side effects of certain allopathic medicines (High Blood Pressure, Heart disease, Kidney diseases, Iron supplements, calcium supplements, narcotics' used to reduce the severe pain)
5. Anxiety, Depression and any other Neurologic disorders
6. Not Enough Activity or exercise
7. Not able to manage your toilet timings or ignoring the urge to pass stools
8. Consuming excess alcohol, smoking and dehydration in the body
9. High levels of estrogen and progesterone during pregnancy may cause constipation

10. Hypothyroidism, or an underactive thyroid gland, slows the body's metabolic processes—even the gut. This may be cause for Constipation.

11. Some Research have found that people have lower back pain are prone to constipation or vice versa. (People with constipation have lower back problems)

5. Complication in Constipation

If you are not able to treat constipation, in the long run you may come across below complications.

1. Piles/Haemorhoids (which can cause pain, itching around anus and swelling of anus. Piles are swollen blood vessels that form in the lower rectum and anus.
2. Faecal Impaction (where dry, hard stools collect in the rectum)
3. Rectal prolapse – This happens when your rectum slips so that it sticks out of your anus. It can happen if you stain during bowel movements. It may cause mucus to leak from your anus.

6. Diagnosis/Tests for Constipation

Blood tests to check on hormone levels

Barium studies to look for any blockages in your colon. For this test, you'll down a special drink and then get an X-ray.

Colonoscopy or other tests to look for blockages in your colon

An Abdominal X-ray where X-ray radiation is used to produce images of the inside of your abdomen

Anorectal manonetry – where a small device with a balloon at one end is inserted into your rectum and attached to a machine that measures and attached to a machine that measures pressure reading from the balloon as your squeeze , relax and push your rectum muscles; this gives an idea of how well the muscles and nerves in and around your rectum are working .

7. Cure for Constipation

There are several methods to cure Constipation without medicines.

Below are the some of the healing techniques used across the world to cure constipation. I am highlighting only Reiki Healing and Relevant Yoga's and Mudra's to Heal Constipation.

1) Reiki Healing

2) Crystal Healing

3) Pranic Healing

4) Mexican Healing

5) Holographic Healing

6) Yoga and Mudra

Reiki Healing for Constipation

A.   Reiki Healing

Reiki is a form of alternative medicine developed in 1922 by Japanese Buddhist Dr. Mikao Usui.

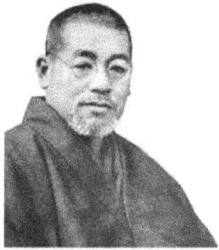

Mikao Usui 臼井甕男 (1865–1926)

It uses a technique commonly called palm healing or hands-on-healing. The word Reiki is made of two Japanese words – Rei which means "God's Wisdom or the Higher Power" and Ki which means "life force energy". So Reiki is actually "spiritually guided life force energy or universal energy".

Constipation can be completely healed using Reiki Healing. Distant Healing (Patients need not be present in the physical location of the healer/Reiki Practitioner) method found to be very effective. Digestive system of human body is controlled by Solar Plexus Chakra within the body. Reiki Healing needs to be passed to the digestive systems and solar plexus chakra for a speedy healing. Reiki healer needs to heal the entire digestive system and metabolic system. With the Reiki, we can set the body clock and timer for passing the stool for life time.

Yoga For Constipation

Yoga is a Sanskrit word meaning "union" and is about getting the mind and the body to work together to find balance, harmony and ultimately better health.Yoga is Physical, mental and spiritual practice or discipline which originated in India. Yoga Gurus from India introduced yoga to the western countries.

In 1980's yoga became popular as a system of physical exercise across the western world. Yoga in Indian Traditions, however is more than physical exercise, it has a meditative and spiritual core.

Yoga can help to calm the mind, which is more important than you probably realize. Constipation can be a constant source of worry and stress for varying different reasons. Yoga can help you to relax (both mentally and physically) and forget any constipation worries through breathing and meditation.

Yoga moves can specifically help ease constipation by stimulating blood flow and energy to your digestive system and its many muscles, which will help to keep peristalsis working, your stools moving more freely through the intestines and, if you are more relaxed, then less likely to strain or cause unwanted pressure in the bowels. With regular practice, yoga could help to keep your digestive system working at its best, and prevent constipation. Below list of yoga's are useful for constipation which you can find in Appendix

1. Mayurasana (Peacock Pose)

2. Ardha Matsyendrasana

3. Halasana (Plough Pose)

4. Pavanmuktasana (Wind-Relieving Pose)

5. Baddha Konasana (Butterfly Pose)

8.Constipation Remedies Summary

In Nut-shell Below are the constipation Remedies Summary you may need to keep in mind.

Food Diet

1. Eat More Vegetables and Include Fiber in your diet
2. Reduce Meat from your daily diet
3. Reduce Oily, fried and fatty foods from your diet
4. Drink 3 Litters of water everyday
5. Reduce Smoking and Alcohol Consumption
6. Avoid those food increases constipation
7. If you are living in the cold countries ensure you get enough fluid food and water during the day time.

Medicines

1. Stop Taking Allopathic Medicines for constipation and other diseases try to switch over to herbal medicines for all your diseases
2. Follow Reiki or other Healing Techniques to replace your Allopathic medicines for the existing chronic diseases. If you have belief in yourself, you can actually cure any diseases.
3. Stop taking Iron or Calcium supplements instead make a habit to consume Iron and Calcium in natural form through green vegetables/seeds/fruits/legumes.

Exercise

1. Conduct those Yoga which stimulate Bowel movements (provided in book)
2. Alternatively ,you can check with your Doctor for suitable exercise which stimulate bowel movements

Life Style Changes

1. Practice Yoga or Meditation to reduce your stress, depression and anxiety levels
2. Practice some stress management techniques to reduce stress level
3. If you have time, practice 7 Chakra Meditation weekly once
4. Practice Mudra for 15 minutes daily or thrice a week
5. Practice some deep breathing exercises helps to stimulate digestion and metabolism
6. Practice Reiki Healing on weekly basis helps you to balance all 7 Chakras which keeps you in good mental and physical health

Appendix A – Food To Be Taken for Constipation

List of Food to be Taken on Daily Basis for Constipation

1   Flax Seeds

2   Beans

3   Broccoli

4   Knolkol

5   Spinach

6   Gram Flour

7   Sweet Potato (Unpeeled) and Watery Vegetable

8   Plums, Prunes, Apples, Kiwis, Oranges, Berries and Papaya

9   Sweet Corn

10   OATS

11   Nuts (Almonds, Peanuts and Walnuts)

12   OKRA /Ladies Finger, Radish

13   Bread Made of Whole Wheat Flour

14   Turmeric, Garlic and Ginger

Appendix B Food To Be Avoided for Constipation

List of Food to be Avoided for Constipation

1   Frozen Snacks, Frozen Foods

2   Processed food such as Hot Dogs, Pizzas, Burgers or some microwavable foods

3   Dairy Products

4   Fried Foods which contain excessive fats

5   Fast Foods

6   Ice Creams and Milkshakes

7   Meat with lot of Iron and Frozen Meats

8   Coffee

9   Alcohol

10 White Flour and Food Made of White Flour

Appendix C Yoga for Constipation

Mayurasana (Peacock Pose)

This posture helps improve digestion and destroys the effects of unwholesome food. It also increases intra-abdominal pressure, which reduces spleen and liver enlargements. The pose is also beneficial in toning the bowels and removing constipation problems.

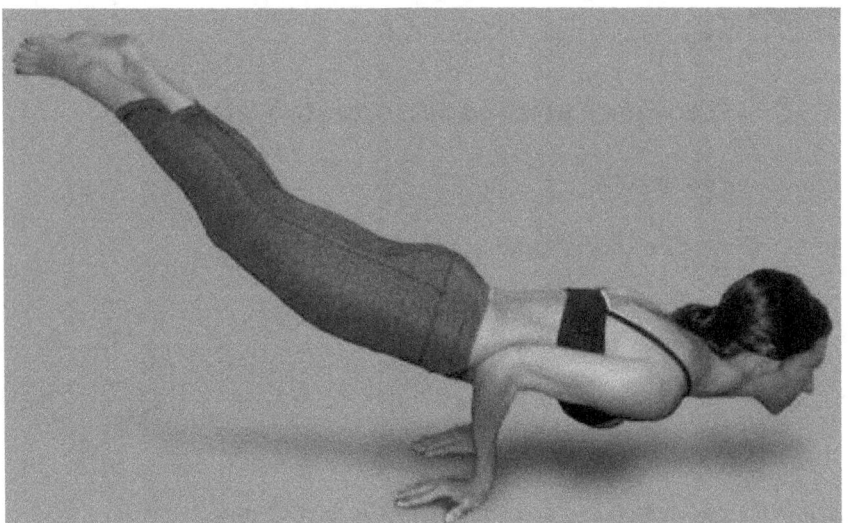

Ardha Matsyendrasana

This asana massages the kidneys, pancreas, small intestines, gall bladder and liver, helping to stimulate digestion and squeeze out   toxins. This yoga is very useful for diabetics, with concentration on the pancreas. It Increases the elasticity of the spine, tones the spinal nerves

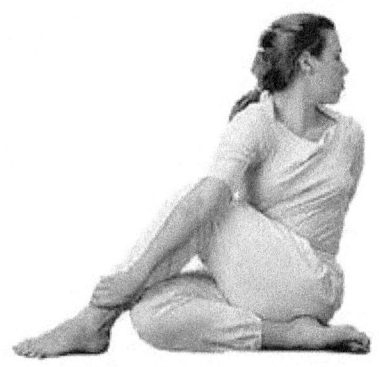

Halasana (Plough Pose)

This posture provides comfort to the liver and intestine. It is an inversion posture which increases blood circulation in the pelvic area and boosts digestion.

It stimulates the pancreas, spleen and activates immune system by massaging all the internal organs including pancreas. It improves kidney and liver functioning and strengthens the abdominal muscles. It also rejuvenates the mind.

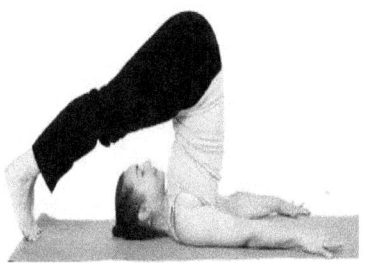

Pavanmuktasana (Wind-Relieving Pose)

As the name suggests, this posture helps release gas from the body, a common trouble for most of us suffering from regular constipation. The posture can help cure several digestive disorders, including dyspepsia. It also helps in relieving acid reflux which is caused by indigestion.

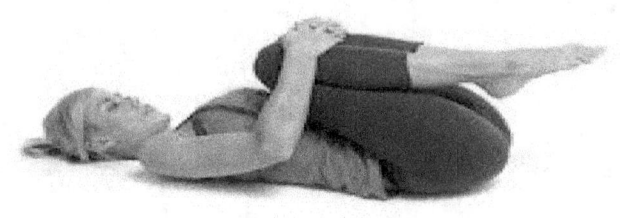

Baddha Konasana (Butterfly Pose)

This forward-bend posture helps improve our digestive system and also relieves gas, cramping and bloating of stomach. The posture also helps in reducing stress which is necessary for good digestion.

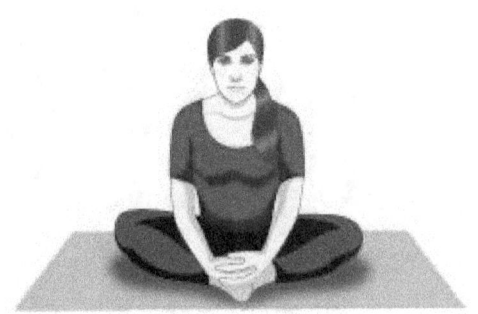

Appendix D Mudra for Constipation

Apan Mudra [Mudra of Digestion]:

This mudra is very useful for curing constipation, piles and diabetes. The mudra, also called the mudra of purification, is one of the easiest yoga mudras. It aids in striking a better balance between the elements within the human body. Thus, it ensures that the unwanted toxins are flushed out properly from your body. This mudra results in frequent urination for eliminating the wastes, thus lowering the blood sugar levels.

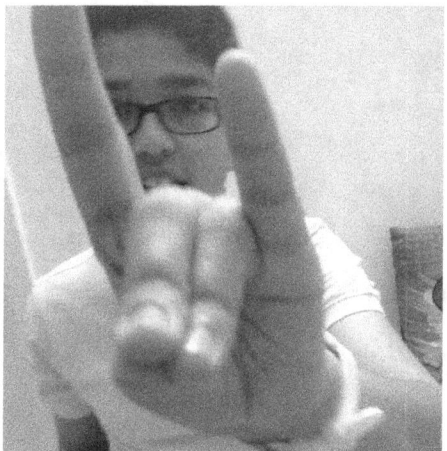

Keeping index finger and ring finger straight, the tip of the thumb should be touched by ring finger and middle finger as seen in the image above.

www.ingramcontent.com/pod-product-compliance
Lightning Source LLC
Chambersburg PA
CBHW072029280526
45788CB00007B/2737